Preface

"In today's fast-paced world, it's easy to fall into unhealthy habits that can take a toll on our bodies. This book is here to help you reclaim your health and vitality through the power of proper nutrition and detoxification. With practical tips, delicious recipes, and a wealth of scientific knowledge, you'll learn how to nourish your body, support your immune system, and rid yourself of toxins that can hold you back from feeling your best."

"From the latest research on nutrition and detoxification to practical strategies for incorporating healthy habits into your daily routine, this book is your guide to optimal health and well-being. Whether you're looking to lose weight, boost your energy, or improve your overall health, you'll find everything you need to start your journey towards wellness in these pages."

"We are constantly bombarded by toxins in our environment, and it's important to give our bodies the support they need to stay healthy and strong. This book is here to help you do just that, with a comprehensive guide to nutrition, detoxification, and healthy living. You'll learn how to nourish your body with wholesome, nourishing foods, and how to support your immune system and eliminate toxins that can hold you back from feeling your best.This book is your roadmap to a happier, healthier life."

Table of Content

Chapter 1 What is Healthy Eating?

Chapter 2: Understanding The Role of Nutrients in our Body

Chapter 3: The role of nutrients in Sports and Exercise Performance

Chapter 9: Individualised Nutritional Planning

9.1 Importance of individualized nutrition planning

9.2 Benefits of Individualized Nutrition Planning

9.3 Sample customized 3 Days meal Plans for weight lifting Athletes, Recovery Support and Weight Loss

9.3 Recipes of Healthy Snacking and Meals

Chapter 1

What is Healthy Eating

Chapter 1   What is Healthy Eating

Eating a healthy diet is an important aspect of overall wellness and can help to prevent chronic diseases such as obesity, heart disease, and diabetes. But what does it mean to have a healthy eating lifestyle?

A healthy eating lifestyle involves more than just making the occasional healthy food choice. It is a long-term pattern of eating that includes a variety of nutritious foods in the right amounts to support good health.

This means choosing a variety of foods from all food groups, including fruits, vegetables, grains, proteins, and dairy. It also means paying attention to portion sizes and being mindful of your overall intake of calories and nutrients.

In addition to the types and amounts of food you eat, a healthy eating lifestyle also involves other factors such as:

- Making time to sit down and enjoy meals without distractions

- Being mindful of your hunger and fullness cues and stopping when you are satisfied

- Limiting your intake of unhealthy foods, such as those high in added sugars, saturated and trans fats, and sodium
- Staying hydrated by drinking plenty of water
- Seeking out sources of reliable nutrition information and staying up to date on the latest recommendations

Adopting a healthy eating lifestyle takes effort and planning, but the benefits are well worth it. By making nutritious food choices and developing healthy habits, you can support your overall health

Chapter 2

Understanding the Role of Nutrients in the Body

Chapter 2: Understanding the Role of Nutrients in the Body

The human body requires a variety of nutrients to function properly and maintain good health. These nutrients can be divided into two main categories: macronutrients and micronutrients.

Macronutrients are nutrients that the body needs in large amounts and include protein, carbohydrates, and fat. These nutrients provide energy and support various functions in the body. Protein is important for the growth, repair, and maintenance of tissues. **Macronutrients and their functions in the body**

2.11Protein is a macronutrient that plays a number of important roles in the body. It is necessary for the growth, repair, and maintenance of tissues such as muscles, skin, and hair. Protein is also important for the production of enzymes, hormones, and other molecules that are involved in various body processes. There are many different sources of protein, including both animal-based and plant-based options. Here are some examples of good sources of protein:

Meat: Beef, chicken, pork, lamb, etc
Poultry: Chicken, turkey, etc.
Fish and seafood: Salmon, tuna, shrimp, etc.
Eggs: Whole eggs or egg whites

Dairy products: Milk, cheese, yogurt, etc.
Beans and legumes: Lentils, chickpeas, kidney beans, black beans, etc.
Nuts and seeds: Almonds, peanuts, sunflower seeds, pumpkin seeds, etc.
Soy products: Tofu, tempeh, edamame, etc.

It is important to consume a variety of protein sources to ensure that you are getting all of the essential amino acids your body needs. It is also important to choose lean sources of protein, such as skinless poultry and fish, and to limit intake of high-fat animal-based proteins, such as fatty cuts of meat and full-fat dairy products.

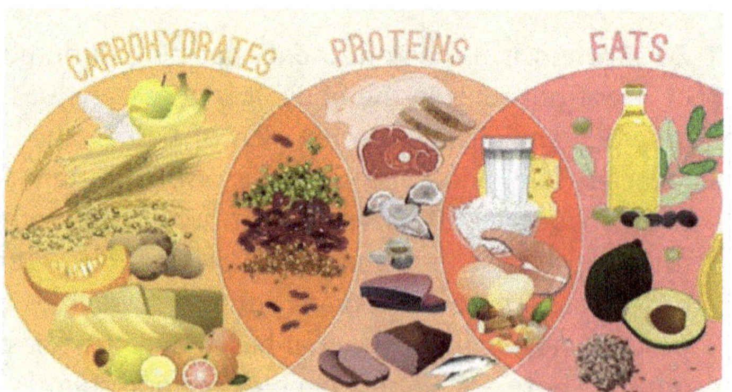

2.12Carbohydrates are another macronutrient that is important for energy production in the body. They are the body's main source of fuel, and can be found in a variety of foods such as grains, fruits, vegetables, and dairy products.

There are two types of carbohydrates:
Simple Carbohydrates   Complex Carbohydrates

<u>What Type of Carbs are healthy to eat and Why?</u>

It's healthy for a body to add more of the complex carbohydrates in meals because Simple carbohydrates, also known as fast-release or high-glycemic index carbs, are absorbed quickly by the body and provide a quick burst of energy. They are found in foods that contain sugar, such as sweets, pastries, and sugary drinks.

Simple carbs can be beneficial in certain situations, such as during exercise when the body needs a quick source of energy. However, consuming too many simple carbs can be harmful to health. They cause a rapid spike in blood sugar levels, followed by a crash in energy. This can lead to feelings of fatigue and can also contribute to weight gain if consumed in excess.

In comparison, complex carbohydrates, also known as slow-release or low-glycemic index carbs, are considered to be better They are absorbed more slowly by the body, which can help to regulate blood sugar levels and provide sustained energy. Complex carbs are typically higher in fiber, which can help to support digestion and may also help to lower cholesterol and blood pressure. Simple carbs are often low in fiber.

In addition, complex carbs are often found in healthier sources of food, such as whole grains, fruits, and vegetables, which are also rich in other important nutrients such as vitamins, minerals, and antioxidants. Simple carbs, on the other hand, are often found in foods such as sugar, sweets, and processed snacks, which are generally low in nutrients.

<u>Some good sources of complex carbs include:</u>

Whole grains: Brown rice, whole wheat, quinoa, oats,

Fruits: Apples, bananas, berries, etc.

Vegetables: Sweet potatoes, peas, corn, etc.

Legumes: Beans, lentils, chickpeas, etc.

2.13 Fat is also a macronutrient that is important for energy production and the absorption of fat-soluble vitamins. It also plays a role in maintaining healthy skin and hair, and protecting the organs. There are different types of fats, including saturated, monounsaturated, and polyunsaturated fats.

Consuming too much **saturated fat** can be dangerous for health because it can raise levels of LDL cholesterol in the blood, which is often referred to as "bad" cholesterol.

High levels of LDL cholesterol can increase the risk of heart disease, which is the leading cause of death worldwide.

Saturated fats can also contribute to other health problems such as obesity and diabetes. They are high in calories and can contribute to weight gain if consumed in excess.

It is generally recommended to limit intake of saturated fats and to choose healthier sources of fat, such as monounsaturated and polyunsaturated fats. These types of fats, which are typically liquid at room temperature, are found in foods such as **avocados, nuts, and olive oil** and may have health benefits such as reducing the risk of heart disease.

Polyunsaturated fats are also typically liquid at room temperature and can be found in foods such as **fatty fish, nuts, and seeds**. They may have health benefits such as reducing the risk of heart disease and lowering cholesterol levels.

There are two types of polyunsaturated fats: **omega-3 fatty acids and omega-6 fatty acids.** Omega-3 fatty acids, which can be found in fatty fish such as salmon, have anti-inflammatory effects and may have benefits for heart health and brain function.

Omega-6 fatty acids, which can be found in vegetable oils, may also have health benefits but are typically consumed in excess in the diet and may contribute to inflammation.

2.1 Micronutrients and their Function in the Body

Micronutrients are nutrients that the body needs in small amounts to function properly. These include vitamins and minerals, which are essential for various functions in the body.

2.21 Vitamins

There are two types of vitamins:

1:water-soluble   2: fat-soluble vitamins.

Water-soluble vitamins, such as vitamin C and the B-complex vitamins, are not stored in the body and must be consumed on a regular basis.

There are nine water-soluble vitamins: vitamin C and the B-complex vitamins (thiamin, riboflavin, niacin, pantothenic acid, vitamin B6, biotin, vitamin B12, and folate).

<u>Vitamin C</u> is important for maintaining healthy skin, tissues, and bones, and it also helps to support the immune system. It can be found in foods such as oranges, strawberries, kiwi, bell peppers, and broccoli.

The <u>B-complex</u> vitamins are important for various functions in the body, such as energy production, nerve function, and the metabolism of carbohydrates, proteins, and fats. They can be found in a variety of foods, including whole grains, meat, poultry, fish, eggs, dairy products, nuts, and seeds.

Unlike fat-soluble vitamins, which are stored in the body, water-soluble vitamins are not stored in the body and must be consumed on a regular basis to ensure that the body has an adequate supply.

Fat-soluble vitamins, such as vitamins A, D, E, and K, are stored in the body and do not need to be consumed as frequently.

Vitamin A can be found in animal-based foods such as liver, eggs, and dairy products, as well as in plant-based sources such as orange and yellow fruits and vegetables.

Vitamin D can be found in fatty fish, eggs, and fortified dairy products, and it can also be synthesized by the body when the skin is exposed to sunlight.

Vitamin E can be found in vegetable oils, nuts, and seeds.

Vitamin K can be found in leafy green vegetables, meat, and dairy products

2.22 Minerals

Minerals are also important for the body. They can be divided into two categories: macro minerals and trace minerals. Minerals have a variety of functions in the body. For example, calcium is important for bone health, iron is necessary for carrying oxygen in the blood, and zinc plays a role in immune function. Here is a list of some important minerals for the body:

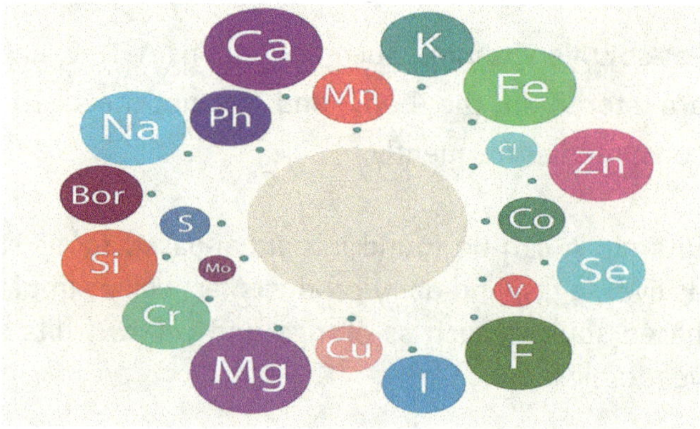

<u>Calcium</u>: important for bone health and muscle function

<u>Sodium:</u> important for fluid balance and nerve function

<u>Potassium</u>: important for heart function and muscle function

<u>Iron</u>: important for carrying oxygen in the blood

<u>Zinc:</u> important for immune function and wound healing

<u>Magnesium</u>: important for bone health and enzyme function

<u>Copper</u>: important for the production of collagen and the absorption of iron

<u>Iodine</u>: important for thyroid function

<u>Selenium</u>: important for thyroid function and antioxidant activity

2.3 The role of fiber in the diet Fiber is a type of carbohydrate that the body cannot digest. It is found in plant-based foods such as fruits, vegetables, whole grains, and legumes.

There are two types of fiber: soluble fiber and insoluble fiber. Soluble fiber dissolves in water and can help to lower cholesterol and blood sugar levels. Insoluble fiber does not dissolve in water and helps to add bulk to the stool, which can support bowel regularity.

Fiber has a variety of roles in the body. It can help to support digestion and prevent constipation, and it may also help to lower cholesterol and blood pressure levels. In addition, fiber can help to regulate blood sugar levels and may assist with weight management.Some good sources of fiber include:

Fruits: apples, berries, oranges, etc.

Vegetables: peas, beans, broccoli, etc.

Whole grains: oats, barley, quinoa, etc.

Legumes: lentils, chickpeas, kidney beans, etc.

There are many seeds that are good sources of fiber, including:

Chia seeds: These small, nutrient-dense seeds are high in fiber, with approximately 11 grams per ounce.

They also contain a good balance of omega-3 and omega-6 fatty acids and are a source of plant-based protein.

Flaxseeds: These seeds are high in fiber, with approximately 8 grams per ounce. They are also a good source of omega-3 fatty acids and contain lignans, which are plant compounds with antioxidant properties.

Hemp seeds: These seeds are high in fiber, with approximately 5 grams per ounce. They are also a good source of plant-based protein and omega-3 and omega-6 fatty acids

Pumpkin seeds: These seeds are high in fiber, with approximately 3 grams per ounce. They are also a good source of minerals such as magnesium and zinc.

Sunflower seeds: These seeds are high in fiber, with approximately 3 grams per ounce. They are also a good source of vitamin E and minerals such as selenium and magnesium.

If the body consumes less fiber, it may experience digestive problems such as constipation. In addition, a diet low in fiber may be associated with an increased risk of certain health problems such as heart disease and diabetes.

There are also supplements that contain fiber, such as psyllium husk and methylcellulose, which can be taken to increase fiber intake. These supplements are often used to treat constipation or to help lower cholesterol levels.However, it is important to note that consuming too much fiber can also have negative effects, such as bloating and gastrointestinal discomfort. It is generally recommended to aim for a moderate intake of fiber, approximately 25-35 grams per day, to support overall health.

2.4 Water and Hyderation?

Water is essential for the proper functioning of the body and is involved in many important processes. It is necessary for the regulation of body temperature, the transportation of nutrients and oxygen to cells, and the removal of waste and toxins from the body.

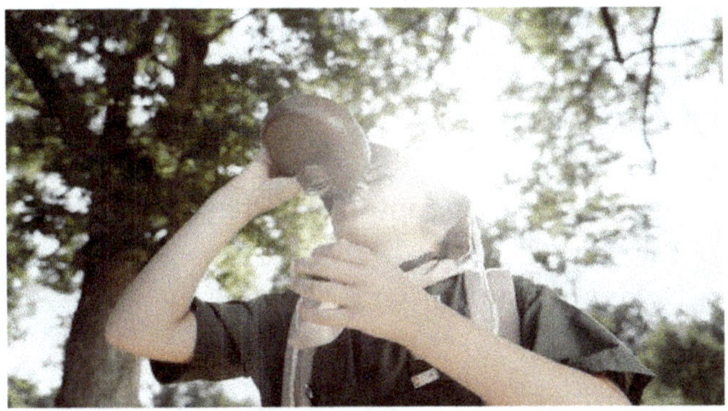

Water makes up a large percentage of the body, and it is important to maintain an adequate level of hydration to support overall health. When the body is dehydrated, it can affect physical and mental performance and can also lead to health problems such as constipation, kidney stones, and fatigue.

It is generally recommended to drink at least 8 cups (64 ounces) of water per day, although individual needs may vary depending on factors such as age, gender, weight, and activity level. Water is the best source of hydration, but it is also found in other beverages and foods, such as fruit and vegetables.

2.41 Symptoms of Dehydrated Body

If you are experiencing any of these symptoms, it is important to drink fluids and rehydrate the body. Water is the best source of hydration, but other beverages such as electrolyte solutions and sports drinks can also help to replenish fluids and electrolytes lost through sweating. Dehydration can range from mild to severe, and it is important to address it as soon as possible to avoid potential health complications.

- Here are some symptoms of dehydration:
- Thirst
- Dry mouth and throat
- Dry, cool skin
- Fatigue or weakness
- Headache
- Dizziness or lightheadedness
- Dark yellow urine
- Dry, sticky mouth and swollen tongue
- Muscle cramps &decreased urine output

If you are experiencing any of these symptoms, it is important to drink fluids and rehydrate the body. Water is the best source of hydration, but other beverages such as electrolyte solutions and sports drinks can also help to replenish fluids and electrolytes lost through sweating.

If you are unable to keep fluids down or if your symptoms are severe, it is important to seek medical attention.

2.42 Tips to Increase Water Intake :

Here are some tips to help you improve your water intake:

- Keep a water bottle with you at all times: Having a water bottle with you makes it easier to remember to drink water throughout the day.

- Drink water with meals: Drinking a glass of water with meals can help to hydrate the body and may also help to fill you up, which can aid in weight management.

- Drink water when you're feeling thirsty: Thirst is a sign that the body is dehydrated, so it is important to drink water as soon as you feel thirsty.

- Drink water before, during, and after exercise: It is important to stay hydrated during physical activity to support performance and recovery.

- Add flavor to your water: If you don't like the taste of plain water, try adding some flavor with sliced fruit or herbs.

- Choose water over sugary drinks: Sugary drinks such as soda and fruit juice can contribute to weight gain and other health problems. Choosing water instead can help to improve hydration and overall health.

- Choose water over sugary drinks: Sugary drinks such as soda and fruit juice can contribute to weight gain and other health problems. Choosing water instead can help to improve hydration and overall health.

- Keep track of your water intake: Using a water tracker app or writing down your water intake can help you to stay on track and ensure that you are meeting your hydration needs.

2.5 Importance of Phyto-chemicals for the Body

Phyto-chemical work in the body in a variety of ways. Some phytochemicals are powerful antioxidants, which means that they can help to reduce oxidative stress and neutralize harmful free radicals in the body. Free radicals are unstable molecules that can damage cells and contribute to the development of chronic diseases, such as cancer and heart disease. By neutralizing free radicals, phytochemicals may help to protect against these diseases and rapid body aging

There are many different types of phytochemicals, including flavonoids, carotenoids, and phytosterols. Each type of phytochemical has its own unique set of health benefits.

Flavonoids are a type of phytochemical that are found in a variety of fruits, vegetables, and other plant-based foods. They are known for their antioxidant properties and have been shown to have a number of potential health benefits, including reducing the risk of heart disease and cancer, and improving cognitive function.

Carotenoids are another type of phytochemical that are found in a variety of fruits and vegetables. They are known for their antioxidant properties and have been shown to have a number of potential health benefits, including reducing the risk of heart disease, cancer, and age-related eye problems.

Phytosterols are a type of phytochemical that are found in a variety of plant-based foods, including nuts, seeds, and vegetable oils. They have been shown to have cholesterol-lowering properties and may help to reduce the risk of heart disease.

.

There are many plant-based foods that are high in phytochemicals and are also edible. Some examples of these foods include: <u>Berries</u>: Berries are a good source of flavonoids and other phytochemicals. They are also high in fiber, vitamins, and minerals, making them a healthy choice for snacks or additions to meals.

<u>Leafy green vegetables</u>: Vegetables such as kale, spinach, and broccoli are high in phytochemicals, including flavonoids and carotenoids. They are also high in vitamins and minerals, making them a nutritious choice for meals and snacks.

<u>Nuts and seeds</u>: Nuts and seeds are a good source of phytosterols and other phytochemicals. They are also high in healthy fats, protein, and other nutrients, making them a nutritious choice for snacks or additions to meals.

<u>Legumes</u>: Legumes, such as beans, lentils, and chickpeas, are high in phytochemicals, including flavonoids and phytosterols. They are also a good

source of protein, fiber, and other nutrients, making them a healthy choice for meals and snacks.

<u>Whole grains</u>: Whole grains, such as whole wheat, oats, and quinoa, are high in phytochemicals and other nutrients, including fiber and minerals. They are a healthy choice for meals and snacks.

It is generally recommended that people consume a variety of plant-based foods to get a wide range of phytochemicals and other nutrients.

2.6 Role of Anti-Oxidants in the Body

Oxidation, a process that occurs in the human body, can harm cell membranes and other structures such as proteins, lipids, and DNA. When the body metabolizes oxygen, it produces unstable molecules known as free radicals. These molecules can steal electrons from other molecules, leading to damage to DNA and other cells.

While the body needs some free radicals to function properly, an excess of free radicals over time can cause irreversible damage and lead to certain diseases, including heart and liver disease, as well as certain types of cancer, such as oral, oesophageal, stomach, and bowel cancer.

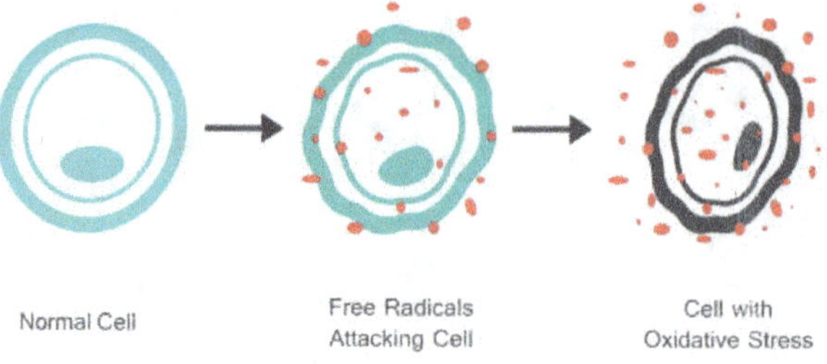

There are various factors that can increase the rate of oxidation in the body, including stress, smoking, alcohol consumption, sunlight exposure, pollution, and more.

Astaxanthin is a pigment that is found in certain seafood, such as salmon, trout, and krill, as well as in some algae. It has been shown to have potent antioxidant properties .It improves body immune system. It may help to protect the skin from the harmful effects of UV radiation.

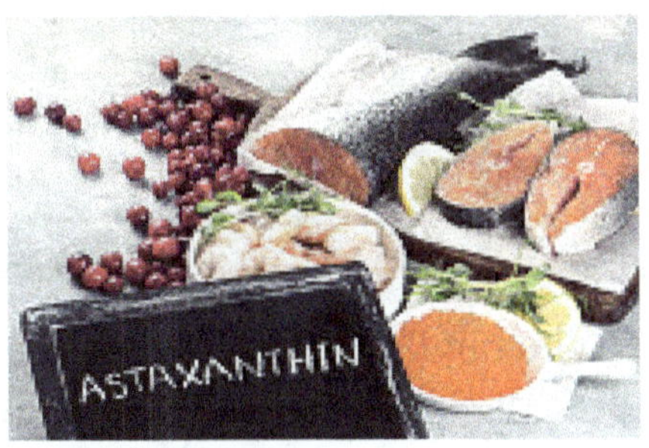

Some research suggests that astaxanthin may help to improve skin moisture, reduce dryness and roughness, and reduce the appearance of wrinkles and improve skin elasticity. However, more research is needed to fully understand the potential benefits of astaxanthin for skin health. It is important to note that while astaxanthin may have some potential benefits for the skin, it is not a replacement for sunscreen and other measures to protect the skin from UV radiation. Astaxanthin also improves eye health by reducing eye fatigue and by promoting capillary blood flow to nourish the eyes.

Vitamin C: Vitamin C is a potent antioxidant that can neutralize free radicals and protect cells from oxidative stress.

It is found in a wide range of fruits and vegetables, including oranges, strawberries, kiwi fruit, bell peppers, and broccoli.

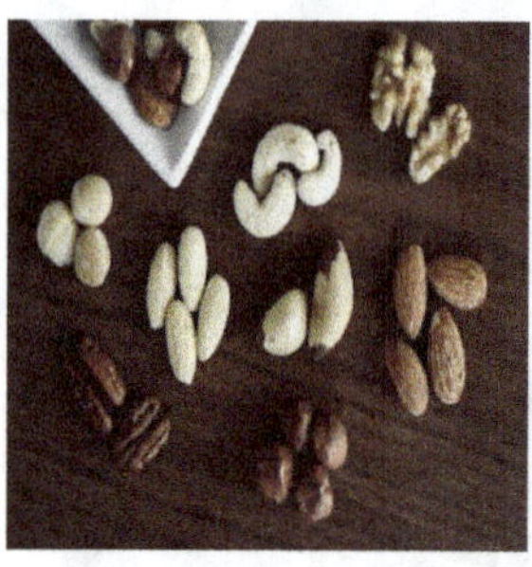 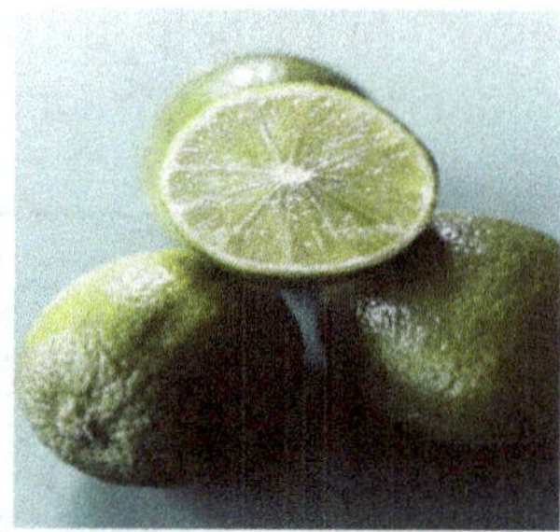

Vitamin E: Vitamin E is another powerful antioxidant that can protect cells from oxidative stress.
It is found in a variety of plant-based oils, nuts, and seeds.

Beta-carotene: Beta-carotene is a carotenoid antioxidant that is converted to vitamin A in the body. It is found in orange and yellow fruits and vegetables, such as carrots, sweet potatoes, and cantaloupe.

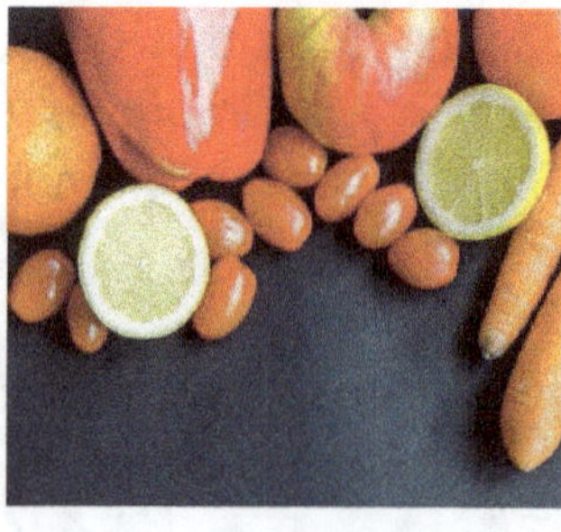 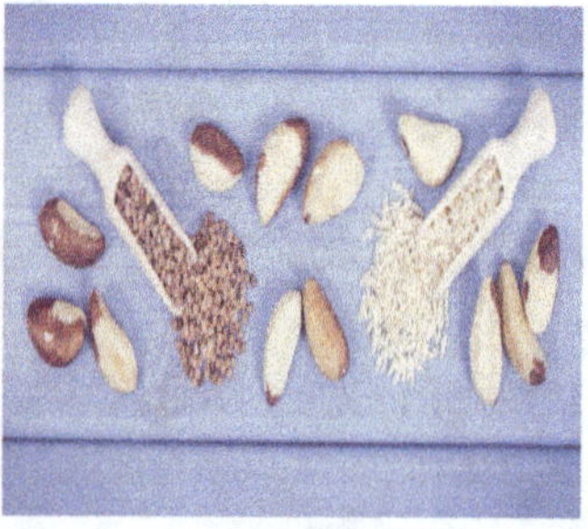

Selenium: Selenium is a trace mineral that is an important component of antioxidant enzymes in the body. It is found in a variety of foods, including Brazil nuts, sunflower seeds, and whole grains.

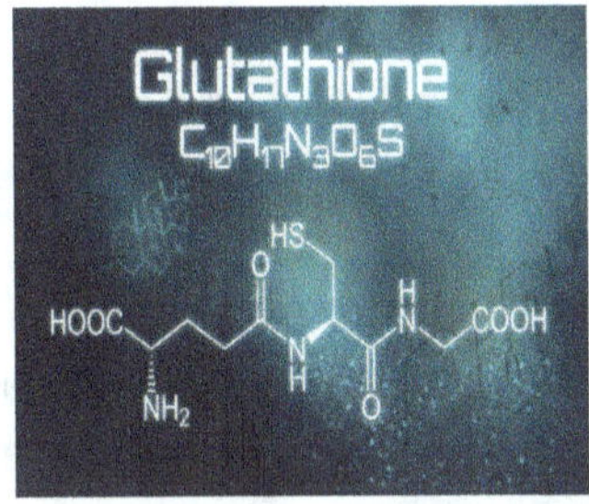

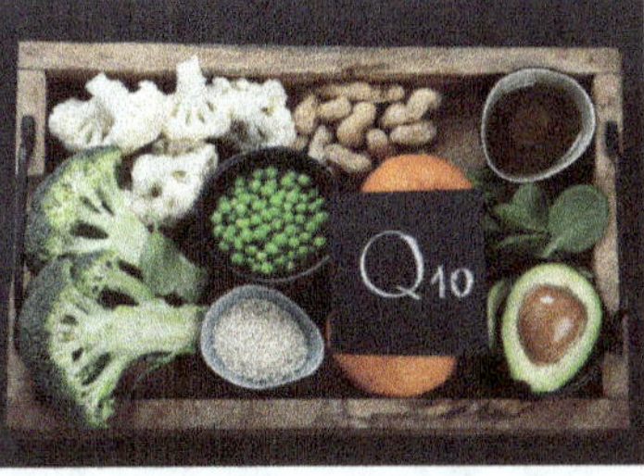

Glutathione: Glutathione is a powerful antioxidant produced by the body that helps to protect cells from oxidative stress. It is found in a variety of foods,including avocados, asparagus, and watermelon.

Coenzyme Q10: Coenzyme Q10 icompound that is involved in energy production in the body and is also a potent antioxidant. It is found in a variety of foods, including fatty fish, organ meats, and whole grains.

Anthocyanins: Anthocyanins are a type of flavonoid antioxidant that is found in a variety of colorful fruits and vegetables, including berries, red grapes, and eggplant.

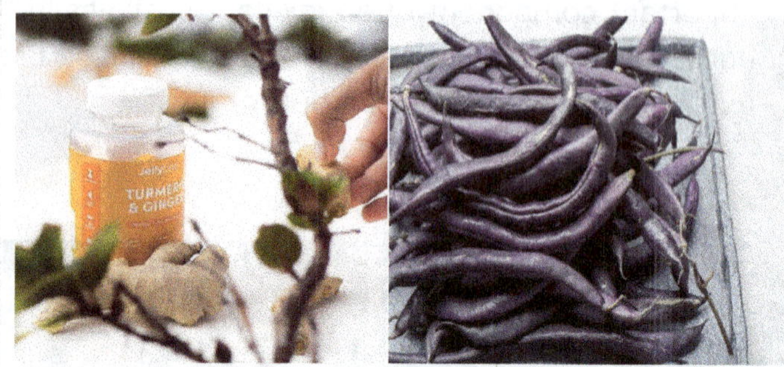

Curcumin: Curcumin is a compound found in turmeric, a spice commonly used in Indian and Middle Eastern cooking. It is a potent antioxidant and has anti-inflammatory properties.

Antioxidants are available in the form of health supplements in market. However its better to get the from food.

2.7 Understanding energy balance and the role of nutrients in weight management

To get fit and active body it is important to keep balance between the energy that you take in through food and beverages, and the energy that you use through physical activity and other body functions.

If you are in energy balance, this means that the energy you take in is equal to the energy you use.

Taken energy = consumed energy (Weight Controlled)

If you are in negative energy balance, this means that you are using more energy than you are taking in, which can lead to weight loss.

Taken Energy < consumed Energy (Weight Loss)

On the other hand, if you are in positive energy balance, this means that you are taking in more energy than you are using, which can lead to weight gain.

Taken Energy > Consumed Energy (Weight Gain)

The role of nutrients in weight management is complex, but in general, the types and amounts of nutrients that you consume can affect your energy balance and your body weight. For example, diets that are high in calories and unhealthy fats may contribute to weight gain, while diets that are high in fiber, lean protein, and healthy fats may help with weight management.

2.71 Energy intake

Energy intake refers to the amount of energy that you take in through food and beverages. The energy content of food is measured in calories. The number of calories that you need depends on your age, sex, weight, height, and physical activity level. Generally, men need more calories than women, and people who are more physically active need more calories than sedentary individuals.

To manage your weight, it is important to be aware of the number of calories that you are consuming. If you are trying to lose weight, you will need to create a **calorie deficit** by taking in fewer calories than you are using. If you are trying to maintain your weight, you will need to be in **energy balance**, which means that the number of calories you consume is equal to the number of calories you use. If you are trying to gain weight, you will need to create a **calorie surplus** by taking in more calories than you are using.

Daily Calories Requirement		
Years	Men	Women
19-30 years	2400-3000 calories	2000-2400 calories
31-59 years	2,200-3,000 calories	1800-2200 calories
60+ Years	2,000-2,600 calories	1600-2000 calories

On the basis of above given chart one can make variations in weight by making changes in the number of calories he takes, depending upon the intensity of weight loss or gain objective, one has decided to achieve.

It is important to note that not all calories are created equal. Different types of foods and beverages have different nutrient profiles, and some are more nutrient-dense than others. Nutrient-dense foods are those that provide a high amount of nutrients (such as vitamins, minerals, and fiber) in relation to their calorie content. For example, vegetables and fruits are generally more nutrient-dense than processed foods that are high in added sugars and unhealthy fats. Choosing nutrient-dense foods can help you to meet your nutrient needs while managing your calorie intake.

Beside making variations in energy one can make varations in energy expenditure to maintaining healthy weight. Here we will find the factors that help in energy expenditure.

2.72 Energy expenditure Energy expenditure refers to the amount of energy that you use through physical activity and other body functions. The energy that you use is measured in calories. The number of calories that you use depends on your age, sex, weight, height, and physical activity level. Generally, men use more calories than women, and people who are more physically active use more calories than sedentary individuals.

To manage your weight, it is important to be physically active and engage in regular exercise. Physical activity can help to increase your energy expenditure, which can help to create a calorie deficit if you are trying to lose weight. It can also help to maintain your weight if you are in energy balance, and can even contribute to weight gain if you are in a calorie surplus.

Physical Activity There are different types of physical activity, including moderate-intensity activities such as brisk walking and cycling, and vigorous-intensity activities such as running and high-intensity interval training. It is generally recommended to aim for at least 150 minutes of moderate-intensity physical activity or 75 minutes of vigorous-intensity physical activity per week, or a combination of both. It is also important to include muscle-strengthening activities at least two days per week.

In addition to physical activity, other factors can affect energy expenditure, including

Non-Exercise Activity Thermogenesis (NEAT)

Resting Metabolic Rate (RMR).

Non-Exercise Activity Thermogenesis (NEAT)
NEAT refers to the energy that you use for activities of daily living such as standing, walking, and fidgeting. It can contribute to your overall energy expenditure and can have an impact on your weight.

For example, people who have high levels of NEAT tend to have a lower body weight, as they are burning more calories through daily activities. On the other hand, people who are sedentary may have lower levels of NEAT and may be at a higher risk of weight gain. Similarly, people who have a high Resting Metabolic Rate RMR tend to burn more calories at rest and may have an easier time maintaining a healthy weight.

Here are some ways to improve NEAT and increase the number of calories you burn through daily activities:

3   Take breaks from sitting: Try to get up and move around every 30 minutes or so, rather than staying seated for long periods of time.

4   Incorporate movement into your daily routine: Find ways to incorporate more movement into your daily routine, such as taking the stairs instead of the elevator, walking or biking to work, or going for a walk during your lunch break.

5   Use a standing desk: Consider using a standing desk or a desk that allows you to stand and work.

6   Do household chores: Incorporate more physical activity into your daily routine by doing household chores such as cleaning, cooking, or gardening.

7   Wear a pedometer or fitness tracker: Wear a pedometer or fitness tracker to track your daily steps and aim to increase your daily step count.

8   Join a sports team or take up a physical hobby: Join a sports team or take up a physical hobby such as dancing or hiking to incorporate more physical activity into your life.

Resting metabolic rate (RMR)

Resting metabolic rate (RMR) refers to the energy that your body uses to perform basic functions such as breathing, circulation, and cell production. People who have a high RMR tend to burn more calories at rest and may have an easier time maintaining a healthy weight.

Here are some ways to improve RMR and increase the number of calories you burn at rest:

1. Build muscle mass: Increasing muscle mass can help to increase RMR, as muscle tissue requires more energy to maintain than fat tissue. Engage in regular strength training and resistance exercises to build muscle mass.

2. Eat enough protein: Consuming adequate amounts of protein can help to increase RMR, as the body requires more energy to digest protein than it does to digest carbohydrates or fat. Aim to include a source of protein in every meal and snack.

3. Stay hydrated: Drinking enough water can help to increase RMR, as the body requires energy to heat cold water to body temperature. Aim to drink at least 8 cups (64 ounces) of water per day.

4. Get enough sleep: Adequate sleep is important for overall health and can also help to increase RMR. Aim for 7-9 hours of sleep per night.

5. Eat enough calories: Consuming too few calories can actually decrease RMR, as the body goes into survival mode and slows down its metabolism to conserve energy. It is important to consume enough calories to support your body's needs and maintain a healthy weight.

Other factors Other factors that can affect energy balance and weight management include:

Stress: Chronic stress can lead to an increase in the stress hormone cortisol, which can affect appetite and metabolism. High levels of cortisol can lead to weight gain, particularly in the abdominal area.

<u>Sleep</u>: Lack of sleep can affect appetite and metabolism, and may increase the risk of weight gain.

<u>Genetics</u>: Some research suggests that genetics can play a role in weight management, as certain genetic factors may influence appetite, metabolism, and the body's ability to store fat.

To effectively manage your weight, it is important to focus on both energy intake and energy expenditure. This can include choosing nutrient-dense foods, engaging in regular physical activity, and finding ways to reduce stress and get enough sleep. It is always a good idea to speak with a healthcare professional for personalized advice on weight management.

2.8 The role of nutrients in immune function

While it is common for people to try to boost their immunity by consuming certain foods or supplements during the flu season or when they are sick, it is important to understand that the immune system is complex and is influenced by a variety of factors, not just diet. While it is true that certain nutrients such as vitamin C and certain foods like citrus fruits, chicken soup, and tea with honey may have immune-boosting properties, they are not a cure-all and cannot replace a healthy, balanced diet and lifestyle. To effectively support immune function, it is important to consume a varied diet that includes a range of vitamins and minerals, and to engage in healthy habits such as getting enough sleep, exercising regularly, and managing stress.

The immune system is a complex network of cells, tissues, and organs that work together to protect the body against harmful substances and microorganisms. It is divided into two main types: **innate immunity and adaptive immunity**. Innate immunity is the first line of defense against pathogens and is achieved through protective barriers such as the skin, mucus, stomach acid, and immune cells that attack foreign cells entering the body.

Adaptive immunity, also known as acquired immunity, is a system that learns to recognize a pathogen and creates specific antibodies and immune cells to attack and destroy it. This system is regulated by cells and organs such as the spleen, thymus, bone marrow, and lymph nodes. Antigens and allergens are substances that can trigger an immune response, while autoimmune disorders and immunodeficiency disorders can depress or disable the immune system.

2.81 Role of microbes in improving immune system

The microbiome refers to the trillions of microorganisms or microbes that live in the body, particularly in the intestines. It is a complex and dynamic field of study, and researchers are discovering that the microbiome plays a vital role in immune function. The gut is a major site of immune activity and the production of antimicrobial proteins. The types of microbes that inhabit the gut can be influenced by diet, particularly a diet that is high in fiber and plant-based foods such as fruits, vegetables, whole grains, and legumes. These types of foods are thought to support the growth and maintenance of beneficial microbes, which can break down fibers into short chain fatty acids that stimulate immune cell activity.

and prebiotic foods may also be beneficial for the microbiome. Probiotic foods contain live helpful bacteria, while prebiotic foods contain fibers and oligosaccharides that nourish and maintain healthy colonies of bacteria. Examples of probiotic foods include kefir, yogurt, fermented vegetables, and kombucha tea, while prebiotic foods include garlic, onions, leeks, and bananas. A general rule for maintaining a healthy microbiome is to consume a variety of fruits, vegetables, beans, and whole grains.

2.82 Role of supplements to improve immune system The role of nutrients in supporting immune function has been studied extensively, and it is well-established that deficiencies in certain nutrients can affect the body's immune response. For example, animal studies have shown that deficiencies in nutrients such as zinc, selenium, iron, copper, folic acid, and vitamins A, B6, C, D, and E can alter immune responses.

These nutrients support immune function in various ways, including acting as antioxidants to protect healthy cells, supporting the growth and activity of immune cells, and helping to produce antibodies. Poor nutrition is also associated with an increased risk of bacterial, viral, and other infections.

While vitamin and herbal supplements may be helpful for addressing specific nutrient deficiencies, it is generally recommended to obtain nutrients through a balanced diet rather than relying on supplements alone.

2.83 Role of herbs to improve immune system

Here are a few herbs that have been traditionally used to support immune function:

Echinacea: Echinacea is a popular herb that is often used to support immune function and reduce the severity and duration of colds and flu. It is thought to stimulate the production of white blood cells and may have antioxidant and anti-inflammatory effects.

Astragalus: Astragalus is an herb that has been used in traditional Chinese medicine to support immune function and reduce the risk of infections. It is thought to stimulate the production of white blood cells and may have antiviral and anti-inflammatory effects.

Ginger: Ginger is a well-known herb that has been used for centuries to support immune function and reduce inflammation. It is thought to have antioxidant and anti-inflammatory properties and may help to reduce the severity and duration of colds and flu.

Garlic: Garlic is a common herb that has been used for centuries to support immune function and reduce the risk of infections.
It is thought to have antimicrobial and antiviral properties and may help to stimulate the production of white blood cells.

Turmeric: Turmeric is a popular herb that has been used for centuries to support immune function and reduce inflammation. It is rich in a compound called curcumin, which has been shown to have antioxidant and anti-inflammatory properties.

2.84 Factors Responsible for Weaken the Immune System

Factors that can weaken the immune system include older age, environmental toxins, excess weight, poor diet, chronic diseases, stress, and lack of sleep. To support immune health, it is important to engage in healthy habits such as eating a balanced diet, exercising regularly, managing stress, and getting enough sleep.

2.9 Nutrients need at different stages of Life

The nutrient needs of an individual change throughout their lifespan as their body undergoes various physical and hormonal changes. Here is an overview of nutrient needs at different stages of life:

<u>Pregnancy</u>: During pregnancy, a woman's nutrient needs are increased as her body is supporting the growth and development of her unborn baby. She will need to consume more folic acid, iron, and calcium, as well as other nutrients such as protein, omega-3 fatty acids, and vitamins D and B6 Folic acid is important for the proper development of the baby's neural tube, which becomes the brain and spinal cord. Adequate intake of folic acid before and during early pregnancy can help prevent major birth defects of the baby's brain and spine.

Iron is needed to produce red blood cells, which carry oxygen to the baby. During pregnancy, a woman's blood volume increases, which means she needs more iron to support the increased blood supply. Without enough iron, a woman can develop anemia, which can lead to fatigue and other health problems.

Calcium is important for the development of the baby's teeth and bones. The baby gets its calcium from the mother, so if the mother does not have enough calcium in her diet, her body will take calcium from her own bones to give to the baby. This can lead to weak bones in the mother.

Protein is important for the growth and repair of tissues in both the mother and the baby.

Omega-3 fatty acids are important for brain and eye development in the baby.

Vitamin D is important for bone health and immune function.

Vitamin B6 is important for the development of the brain and nervous system in the baby. It is also needed to help the body use and store energy from protein and carbohydrate Infancy: Infants have very high nutrient needs due to their rapid growth and development. They require a diet that is rich in breast milk or formula, which provides all the nutrients they need. As they transition to solid foods, they will need to consume a variety of nutrient-dense foods, including iron-rich foods such as meat, fish, and beans, and calcium-rich foods such as milk, cheese, and yogurt.

Childhood: As children grow and develop, their nutrient needs continue to change. They will need to consume a varied diet that includes a balance of protein, carbohydrates, healthy fats, and a wide range of vitamins and minerals. It is important for children to get enough fiber, iron, and calcium to support their growth and development.

Adolescence: During adolescence, both boys and girls experience rapid growth and hormonal changes that affect their nutrient needs. They will need to consume more calories and protein to support their growth and development, as well as increased amounts of certain nutrients such as iron, calcium, and zinc.

Adulthood: In adulthood, nutrient needs generally remain stable. However, adults may have higher or lower nutrient needs depending on factors such as their gender, size, age, and level of physical activity. It is important for adults to consume a balanced diet that includes a variety of nutrient-dense foods, as well as to get enough vitamins and minerals to support their overall health.

Older age: As people age, their nutrient needs may change due to factors such as a decrease in appetite, changes in metabolism, and an increased risk of certain health conditions. Older adults may need to consume more protein, as well as increased amounts of certain vitamins and minerals such as vitamin D and B12. It is important for older adults to consume a healthy and varied diet to support their overall health and well-being.

2.10 The Impact of Environmental Condition and its effect on Nutritional Needs of Athletes

Environmental conditions can have a significant impact on an athlete's nutrient needs. For example:

Altitude: At high altitudes, the body may require more oxygen to function properly, leading to an increased need for carbohydrates to fuel the body. Additionally, the body may lose more fluids through sweat due to the dry air, leading to an increased need for hydration.

Heat: In hot weather, the body may lose more fluids through sweat, leading to an increased need for hydration. It is also important to replace electrolytes lost through sweat, such as sodium and potassium.

Cold: In cold weather, the body may require more calories to maintain body temperature, leading to an increased need for carbohydrates and fats. It is also important to stay hydrated, as the body can lose fluids through respiration in cold air.

Humidity: High humidity can increase sweat loss and lead to an increased need for hydration. It is also important to replace electrolytes lost through sweat.

Athletes competing in extreme environmental conditions may need to adjust their nutrition and hydration strategies to meet their increased needs. It is important for athletes to work with a registered dietitian or nutritionist to create a personalized nutrition plan that takes into account their specific needs and goals.

Chapter 3

Nutrients Need in Athletes and Exercise Performance

Chapter 3 Nutrients Need in Athletes and Exercise Performance

People who regularly do sports or exercise, definitely need more calories and nutrient dense diet as compared to the people who are less involved in these activities. Here are the few important tips.

3.1 keeping the Body Hydrated

When the body is properly hydrated, it is able to function at its optimal level and perform at its best. However, if an athlete is dehydrated, their performance can suffer.

Dehydration can lead to fatigue, muscle cramps, and impaired concentration and decision making. It can also negatively impact thermoregulation, leading to increased body temperature and increased risk of heat stroke.

Proper hydration is especially important for endurance athletes, as they may lose significant amounts of fluids through sweat during long periods of exercise.

It is important for these athletes to replace fluids regularly during exercise to maintain optimal performance.

Additionally, the type of fluid an athlete consumes can impact their hydration status. Water is the most important fluid for hydration, but sports drinks with electrolytes can also be beneficial for endurance athletes to help replace lost electrolytes.

In summary, proper hydration is essential for optimal sports and exercise performance, and athletes should prioritize staying hydrated before, during, and after exercise.

3.2 Impact of over and under Nutritious diet on athletes

Over-nutrition, or consuming more calories than the body needs, can lead to weight gain and decreased athletic performance. Excess body fat can increase the workload on the body during exercise, leading to increased fatigue and decreased endurance. Additionally, over-nutrition can increase the risk of developing health problems such as obesity, diabetes, and heart disease.

Under-nutrition, or consuming too few calories, can also negatively impact sports and exercise performance. A lack of sufficient calories can lead to decreased muscle mass, decreased strength and endurance, and impaired recovery from exercise. Under-nutrition can also compromise the immune system, making athletes more susceptible to illness and injury.

It is important for athletes to consume a balanced diet that provides the necessary nutrients to fuel their workouts and support recovery. Individualized nutrition planning can help athletes achieve optimal performance and prevent over- or under-nutrition.

3.3 Nutritional Properties for Pre-Post Exercise Meals

Proper nutrition is essential for optimal sports and exercise performance, and strategic meal planning can help athletes fuel their workouts and support recovery. Here are some tips for pre- and post-exercise meals:

Pre-exercise meals

- Consume a meal or snack 1-3 hours before exercise to provide energy and fuel for the workout.
- Choose foods high in carbohydrates, such as whole grains, fruits, and vegetables, to provide energy.
- Include a source of protein, such as lean meat, dairy, or plant-based protein sources, to support muscle repair and recovery.
- Avoid high-fat foods, as they can slow digestion and lead to discomfort during exercise.
- Stay hydrated by drinking water or a sports drink before and during exercise.

Post-exercise meals:

- Consume a meal or snack within 30-60 minutes after exercise to support recovery and replenish glycogen stores.

- Choose foods high in carbohydrates to help replenish glycogen stores and restore energy levels.
- Include a source of protein to support muscle repair and recovery.
- Stay hydrated by drinking water or a sports drink.
- Consider incorporating a sports drink with electrolytes to help replace any lost electrolytes during exercise.

It is important to note that individual needs and goals will vary, and it may be necessary to work with a registered dietitian or nutritionist to create a personalized nutrition plan.

3.4 Foods for preventing and recovering Injury

Proper nutrition is important for preventing injury in athletes. Here are some specific foods that can help support injury prevention:

Fruits and vegetables: These foods are rich in antioxidants and nutrients that can help support overall health and immune function, reducing the risk of illness and injury.

Lean protein sources: Adequate protein intake is important for maintaining and repairing muscles, helping to prevent muscle strains and tears.

Examples of lean protein sources include chicken, fish, tofu, and legumes.

Whole grains: Whole grains provide complex carbohydrates and fiber, which can help support energy levels and prevent muscle fatigue.

Water: Adequate hydration is important for maintaining optimal body function and reducing the risk of muscle cramps and heat-related injuries.

Calcium-rich foods: Calcium is important for maintaining strong bones and reducing the risk of fractures. Foods rich in calcium include dairy products, leafy green vegetables, and fortified foods.

Moreover there are certain herbs and foods may help support injury recovery. Here are a few examples:

Turmeric: Turmeric is a spice that contains curcumin, which has anti-inflammatory properties and may help reduce inflammation and pain associated with injury. Turmeric can be consumed in the form of a supplement or added to foods as a spice.

Ginger: Ginger is a herb that also has anti-inflammatory properties and may help reduce inflammation and pain associated with injury. Ginger can be consumed in the form of a supplement or added to foods as a spice.

Collagen: Collagen is a protein that helps support the structure and function of tissues, including bones, muscles, and skin. Supplementing with collagen may help support injury recovery and repair. Bone broth, chicken and fish are good sources of collagen.

Protein-rich foods: Adequate protein intake is important for maintaining and repairing tissues, including muscles, bones, and skin. Examples of protein-rich foods include chicken, fish, tofu, and legumes.

Omega-3 fatty acids: Omega-3 fatty acids are polyunsaturated fats that have anti-inflammatory properties and may help reduce inflammation and pain associated with injury. Omega-3 fatty acids can be found in foods such as fatty fish, nuts, and seeds.

Chapter 4

How to Create a Balanced Diet?

Chapter 4   How to Create a Balanced Diet?

1. Include a variety of foods: A balanced diet includes a variety of foods from all food groups, including fruits, vegetables, grains, protein sources, and dairy (or alternative sources of calcium).

2. Focus on whole, unprocessed foods: Choose whole, unprocessed foods as much as possible, such as whole grains, fruits, vegetables, and lean protein sources. These foods are generally more nutrient-dense and less processed, providing more health benefits.

3. Choose healthy fats: Choose healthy fats, such as monounsaturated and polyunsaturated fats, over unhealthy fats, such as saturated and trans fats. Good sources of healthy fats include olive oil, avocados, nuts, and seeds.

4. Pay attention to portion sizes: Portion sizes are important for maintaining a balanced diet. Be mindful of how much you are eating and aim to balance your intake of different food groups.

5. Consider your individual needs and goals: Everyone has different nutrient needs based on factors such as age, gender, weight, and activity level. Consider consulting with a registered dietitian or nutritionist to create a personalized nutrition plan that meets your specific needs and goals.

6. Considering individual need and goals, supplements can be added. Specially water soluble vitamins can be added. However to add fat soluble vitamins one must take precautionary measures by going through body requirement tests for vitamins.

4.1 Recommended Portions of Food in a plate

A balanced diet can be visualized using the food plate model, which recommends dividing your plate into four quarters

1quarter: Grains (such as whole grain bread, pasta, or rice)

-1quarter: Protein (such as chicken, fish, tofu, or legumes

-2 quarters: Vegetables and fruits (a variety of colors and types)

-1 serving: Dairy (or alternative sources of calcium)

4.2 Examining Food Labels and Reading Serving Size

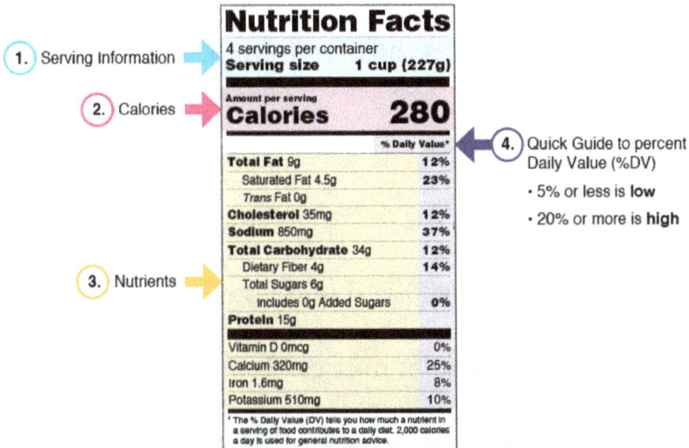

Step 1: Check the serving size The serving size listed on the label is the reference amount of the food that is used to calculate the nutrients listed on the label. Make sure to compare the serving size to the amount you are actually consuming.

Step 2: Look at the calorie content The label will list the number of calories per serving size. Use this information to determine if the food fits into your daily caloric needs. Remember, if you consume more than one serving, you will need to multiply the number of calories by the number of servings you consume.

Step 3: Review the nutrient content The label lists the amount of nutrients per serving size, including fat, cholesterol, sodium, carbohydrates, fiber, and protein. This can help you determine if the food is a good source of a particular nutrient.

Step 4: Consider the % Daily Value (%DV)

The % Daily Value (%DV) tells you how

 much of a particular nutrient is in one

serving of the food in relation to the

recommended daily amount. For example,

if a food has a %DV of 20% for sodium,

it means that one serving of the food

contains 20% of the recommended daily

 amount of sodium.

Step 5: Examine the ingredient list The ingredients are listed in descending order by weight. This means that the first ingredient listed makes up the largest portion of the food.

The percent Daily Values (DV) can be used as a guide to help evaluate how a particular food fits into your daily meal plan. The %DV is based on the average daily nutrient needs of a person consuming 2,000 calories per day and is applicable to an entire day, not just one meal or snack. For example, a food item with a 5% DV of fat provides 5% of the total fat that a person who needs 2,000 calories per day should eat.

	% Daily Value*
Total Fat 9g	**12%**
Saturated Fat 4.5g	**23%**
Trans Fat 0g	
Cholesterol 35mg	**12%**
Sodium 850mg	**37%**
Total Carbohydrate 34g	**12%**
Dietary Fiber 4g	**14%**
Total Sugars 6g	
Includes 0g Added Sugars	**0%**
Protein 15g	
Vitamin D 0mcg	0%
Calcium 320mg	25%
Iron 1.6mg	8%
Potassium 510mg	10%

It is important to note that individual caloric needs may be different from the average person. This means that you may need more or less than the 100% DV listed on the package for certain nutrients. It is recommended to aim for foods that are low in saturated fat, trans fat, cholesterol, and sodium, and high in vitamins, minerals, and dietary fiber. However, it is important to include a variety of foods in your diet and not to focus on any single nutrient in isolation. A healthy diet should include a balance of nutrients from different food groups.

4.3 Understand the Nutrition Terms

Nutrition terms can help you make informed choices about the foods you eat. Here are some common nutrition terms and what they mean:

Low calorie: A food with 40 calories or less per serving is considered low calorie.

Low cholesterol: A food with 20 milligrams or less of cholesterol and 2 grams or less of saturated fat per serving is considered low in cholesterol.

Reduced: A food that contains at least 25% less of a specified nutrient or calories than the usual product is considered reduced.

Good source of: A food that provides at least 10-19% of the Daily Value (DV) of a particular vitamin or nutrient per serving is considered a good source of that nutrient.

Excellent source of: A food that provides at least 20% or more of the DV of a particular vitamin or nutrient per serving is considered an excellent source of that nutrient.

Calorie free: A food that contains less than 5 calories per serving is considered calorie free.

Fat free/sugar free: A food that contains less than ½ gram of fat or sugar per serving is considered fat free or sugar free.

Low sodium: A food with 140 milligrams or less of sodium per serving is considered low in sodium.

High in: A food that provides 20% or more of the DV of a specified nutrient per serving is considered high in that nutrient.

Chapter 5

Preparing and Planning Meals

Chapter 5. Preparing and Planning Healthy Meals

Planning and preparation of healthy meals requires consideration of many factors including age specified goals, budget, weather, cooking style and so on. Here are few tips that will definitely help you in preparing better meal to improve your physical and mental health.

5.1 Determine Nutritional Needs

Measure the height and weight of the patient. Body mass index (BMI) calculated from these variables can help determine whether you are undernourished or over nourished.

$$BMI = \frac{Weight\ (Kg)}{(Height\ in\ metres)^2}$$

$$OR$$

$$BMI = \frac{703 \times Weight\ (lb)}{(Height\ in\ inches)^2}$$

BMI	Weight status
Below 18.5	Underweight
18.5-24.9	Normal weight
25.0-29.9	Overweight
30.0-34.9	Obesity class I
35.0-39.9	Obesity class II
Above 40	Obesity class III

Finding BMI as per given formulae can help determining if you are underweight, ideal weight, overweight or obese.

Find Nutritional Requirements of Your Body. Under weight people usually have nutritional deficiencies but often overweight, obese and normal weight people finds nutritional deficiencies. Nutritionaly deficient body shows few symptoms which works as alarm to inform us.

Symptoms of nutritional deficiency can vary depending on the specific nutrient involved and the severity of the deficiency. Some common symptoms of nutritional deficiency include:

Fatigue
Weakness /Weight loss
Poor appetite
Dry, thinning hair
Dry, rough, scaly skin
Brittle nails
Swelling in the legs
Irritability
Cognitive difficulties

If you are experiencing any of these symptoms, it is important to speak with a healthcare professional to determine the cause and receive appropriate treatment. It is also important to note that these symptoms can be caused by a variety of other factors and may not necessarily be due to a nutritional deficiency.

5.2: Some Clinical Tests to Help Identifying Nutritional Requirements

There are several clinical tests that can help a person understand their nutritional requirements:

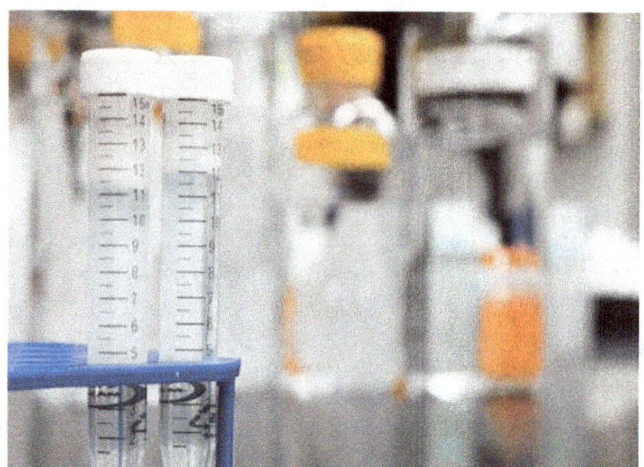

However it is necessary to consult healthcare professional.

1.**Blood tests: Blood** tests can measure the levels of various nutrients in the body, such as vitamins, minerals, and amino acids. This can help identify any deficiencies or imbalances that need to be addressed through diet or supplements.

2. **Body composition analysis:** Techniques such as dual-energy x-ray absorptiometry (DXA) or bioelectrical impedance analysis (BIA) can measure the percentage of fat, muscle, and bone in the body. This can help determine if a person's weight is within

a healthy range and if they are getting enough protein to support muscle mass.

3. Food diary analysis: Keeping a food diary can help a person understand their current eating habits and identify any areas where they may be falling short on nutrients. A healthcare professional can analyze the diary to recommend dietary changes.

4. Nutritional assessment: A comprehensive nutritional assessment typically includes a combination of the above tests, as well as a physical exam, medical history review, and possibly other tests (e.g., blood pressure, cholesterol). This can give a comprehensive picture of a person's nutritional status and help determine any necessary dietary changes.

5. Food intolerance tests: These tests can identify if a person has an intolerance or sensitivity to certain foods. Avoiding these foods can help improve symptoms and overall health.

5.3 Tips for Making a Grocery List of Healthy Foods

Once you calculated your BMI and analyzed your body health condition generally through guidelines given above, it is required from you to decide the goal you want to achieve consider your present health and your dream body shape n size. After that make a list of grocery items that you require.

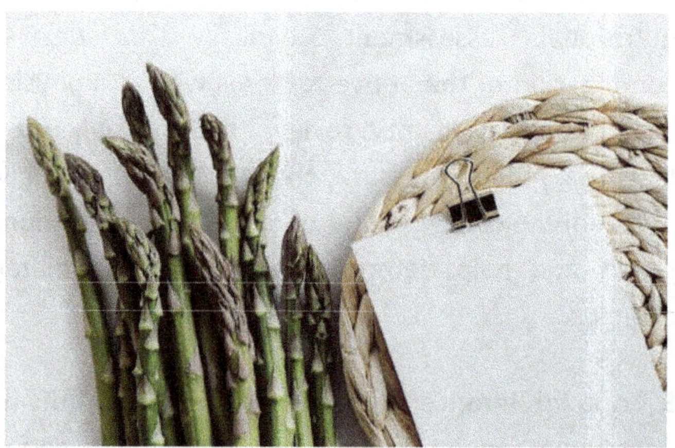

Here are some tips for making a grocery list of healthy foods:

1. Determine your nutritional needs: Consider your age, gender, weight, height, and physical activity level to determine what types and quantities of foods you need to support your health.

2. Choose whole, unprocessed foods: Focus on selecting foods that are minimally processed and close to their natural state, such as fruits, vegetables, whole grains, and lean proteins.
3. Make a list of staples: Make a list of the staple foods that you regularly use in your meals and snacks, such as oats, rice, beans, nuts, and seeds.
4. Plan your meals and snacks: Think about what meals and snacks you'll be preparing for the week and make a list of the ingredients you'll need. This will help you stay organized and avoid last-minute, unhealthy choices.
5. Consider food allergies and intolerances: If you have any food allergies or intolerances, make sure to include alternative options on your list.
6. Don't forget about healthy fats: Healthy fats, such as avocado, olive oil, and nuts, butter and traditional grass fed organic ghee are an important part of a healthy diet. Make sure to include these on your list as well.
7. Be mindful of portion sizes: Consider the portion sizes you'll need for your meals and snacks and make sure to include the appropriate amounts on your list.
8. Add protein sources in your list. Add animal protein sources meat, chicken, fish eggs . Add plant based sources of protein like a variety of seeds and nuts.

Chapter 6

Why We Age ?

Chapter 6: Aging Process can be Slowed Down

6.1 Why We age?

Aging is a natural process that occurs over time as a result of various factors, including genetics and environmental influences. As we age, the body goes through a number of changes, including a decline in physical and cognitive function.

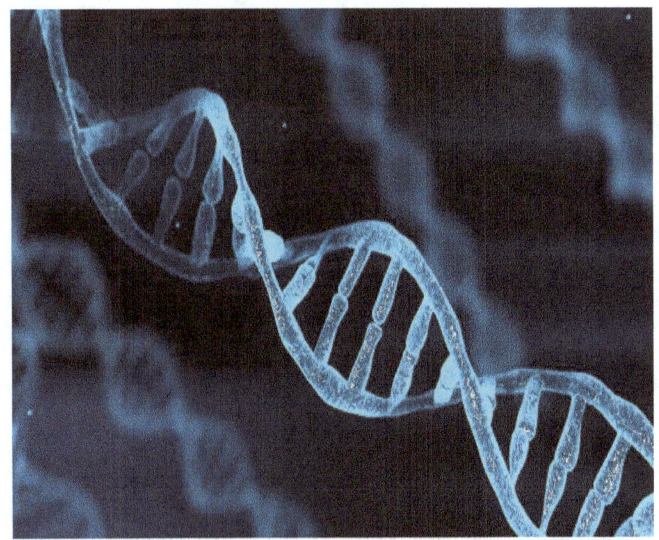

These changes are thought to be caused by a number of factors, including:

Slow metabolism: A slow metabolism can make it more difficult for the body to eliminate toxins, which can lead to an accumulation of toxins in the body.

This can increase the production of free radicals, which can cause DNA damage.

Free radicals: Free radicals are unstable molecules that can cause damage to cells and DNA. They can be generated by toxins, radiation, and other environmental factors.

DNA damage: DNA damage can be caused by a variety of factors, including free radicals, toxins, radiation, and certain medications. DNA damage can lead to mutations and other changes in the DNA molecule, which can affect the normal function of cells.

The accumulation of DNA damage: Over time, cells in the body accumulate damage to their DNA, which can affect their function and contribute to the aging process.

Other Factors that contribute to aging

<u>Decreased hormone production</u>: As we age, the body's production of certain hormones, such as estrogen(female sex hormone) and testosterone(male sex hormone), begins to decline, which can lead to changes in the body and affect the aging process.

<u>Inflammation:</u> Chronic inflammation has been linked to a number of age-related diseases and may contribute to the aging process.

<u>Oxidative stress</u>: The body is exposed to a number of sources of oxidative stress, such as pollution and UV radiation, which can cause damage to cells and contribute to the aging process

Overall, DNA damage plays a significant role in the aging process and the development of various diseases, and it is important to take steps to reduce the risk of DNA damage occurring.

6.2 How to Slowdown Aging Process?

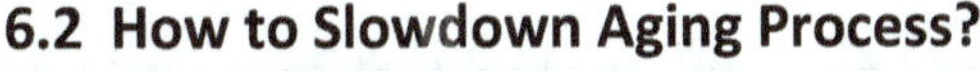

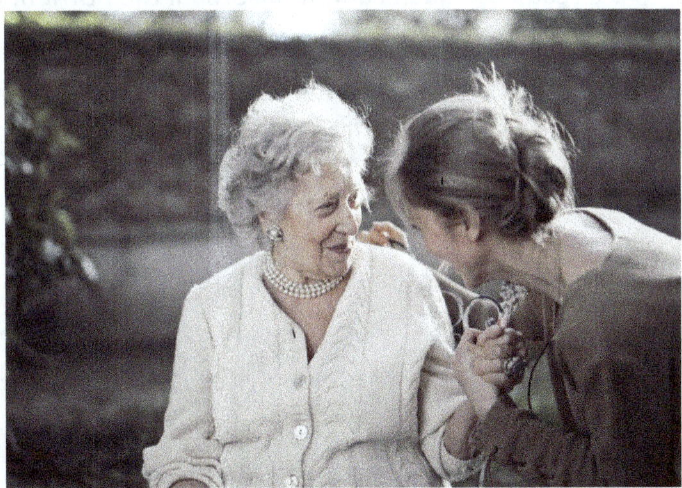

While it is not possible to completely stop the aging process. However there are certain factors that can help us slow down the aging process by reducing DNA damage.

6.21 Steps to Maintain Gut health As we age, the gut microbiome changes, and the diversity of bacteria can decrease. This can lead to an imbalance of the microbiome, which can contribute to various health problems, such as digestive issues, diarrhea constipation . Also when we eat unhealthy calories dense high sugar, carb and fat diet, it reduces our stomach acid which reduces our ability to digest food.

 As a result stomach cannot absorb all the nutrients from food that we eat, no matter how nutritionally dense food you eat if stomach is weak , your body's power to fight against free radicals decreases which leads to DNA damage and sickness.

There are many other factors which destroy the gut health. These are described in the picture given below.

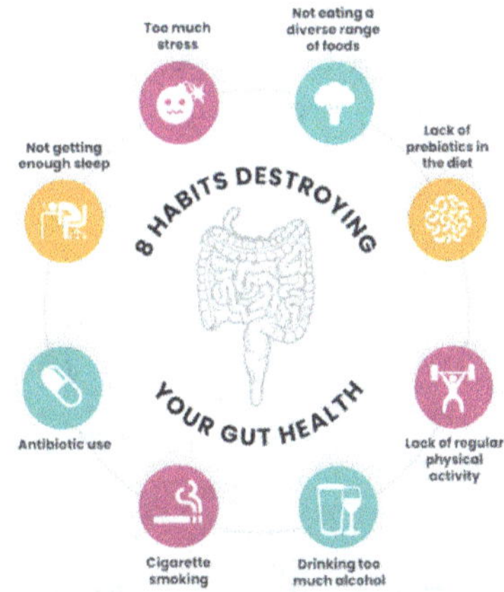

Here are the few tips to maintain gut health:

1. Add fermented food in your diet

Incorporate fermented foods into your diet: Fermented foods, such as yogurt, kefir, and sauerkraut, contain pro-biotic, which are beneficial bacteria that can help promote a healthy gut microbiome. Probiotics are live microorganisms that are similar to the beneficial microorganisms found in the human gut. They are often referred to as "good" or "helpful" bacteria because they help keep the gut healthy.

Probiotics are available in supplements and foods, such as <u>yogurt</u> and <u>fermented vegetables</u>. They are thought to have a number of health benefits, including improving digestion, boosting the immune system, and preventing the growth of harmful bacteria.

2. Use Pro-biotic Supplements

Take pro-biotic supplements for a month to improve stomach health.

3. Use Organic Apple Cider Vinegar

Take 1 to 2 tablespoons of apple Cider Vinegar diluted in water every day early morning. It will increase stomach acid whichwill help with digestion.

6.3 Improve Metabolism:

- Eat smaller more frequent meals
- Take protein rich food. It has high thermal effect.
- Incorporate spicy foods in your diet.
- Avoid sugary drinks and snacks
- Avoid crash diets
- There are certain foods /herbs which improve metabolism. Green tea, ginger, turmeric, garlic, lemon Cruciferous vegetables: apple cider Vinegar

6.4 Inflammation Reasons Symptoms and Ways to reduce it

One of the biggest reason of fast ageing process is body inflammation. Autoimmune diseases, environmental factors, allergies stress and highly processed with high fats and sugar content leads to body inflammation.

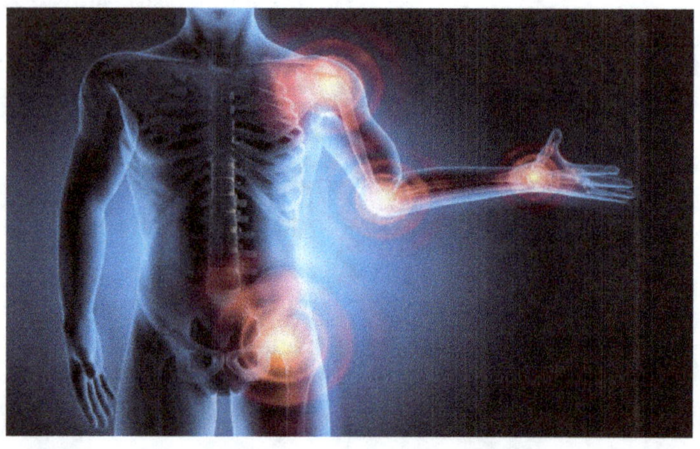

6.41 Symptoms and suggestions to improve Body Inflammation

There are number of signs that indicate that body is suffering from inflammation e.g. pain, swelling, redness, loss of function of affected area, fatigue and weight changes.

 Here are a few tips that may be helpful maintaining health by keeping you away from stress as well as reducing body inflammation and body toxicity.

Exercise regularly: Exercise has been shown to reduce stress and improve overall well-being.

Get plenty of sleep: Adequate sleep is important for managing stress and maintaining overall health.

Practice relaxation techniques: Techniques such as deep breathing, meditation, and yoga can help to reduce stress and promote relaxation.

Take breaks and practice self-care: Set aside time for activities that you enjoy and that help you relax, such as reading, listening music, spending time with friends and loved ones, or taking a walk in nature.

Eat a healthy diet: A diet that is rich in fruits, vegetables, and other nutrients can help to support overall health and well-being.

Detox your body

1. Seek support: Talking to a trusted friend or loved one, or seeking the support of a mental health professional, can be helpful for managing stress.

2. Set boundaries: It is important to set limits and say no to commitments that are not realistic or that add unnecessary stress to your life.

3. Practice gratitude: Focusing on the things that you are grateful for can help to reduce stress and improve your overall outlook on life.

6.5 Body Organs Detox

Detoxification is the process by which the body removes toxins 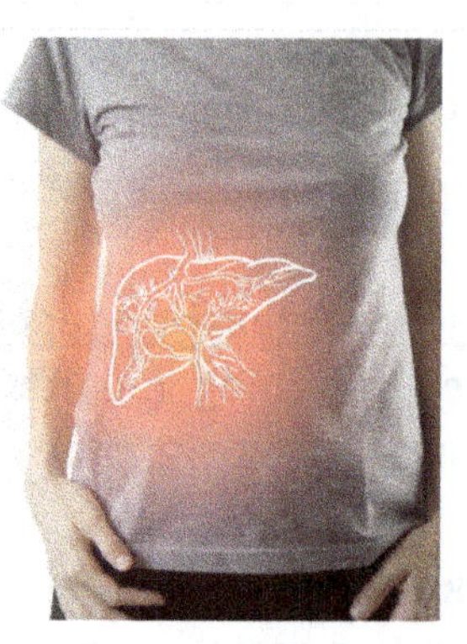 that have accumulated from the environment, diet, and lifestyle. Detoxification is important for maintaining overall health and wellness because it helps to support the body's natural processes for eliminating toxins and waste products.

There are several systems in the body that contribute to detoxification, including the liver, kidneys, and colon. These systems work together to filter out and eliminate toxins from the body. When the body is overloaded with toxins, it can become less efficient at eliminating them, which can lead to a build-up of harmful substances in the body.

This build-up can potentially lead to a range of health problems, including fatigue, digestive issues, skin problems, and even more serious conditions.

Detox Your Liver

Toxicity of liver due to consumption of tobacco, high carbs and sugary foods, frequent body inflammation, chemical sprayed vegetables and fruits, processed food and unhealthy gut 80 % of role in speedy ageing. Other than exercise, good sleep and healthy eating there are a varity of food items that can help detoxifying liver for instance leafy green vegetables have good amount of glutathione, vitamin C, folate chlorophyll and vitamin K which play active role in liver detoxification. One must take a bowl full of green leafy vegetable every day to remove liver toxins. Garlic, turmeric, avocados and nuts are also effective for marinating liver health.

Supplements for Quick Liver Detoxification:

There are several supplements that are claimed to support liver detoxification and improve liver health. These include milk thistle, N-acetyl cysteine (NAC), and alpha-lipoic acid.

Milk thistle is a herb that has been traditionally used to support liver health. It contains a compound called silymarin, which is thought to have antioxidant and anti-inflammatory effects.

N-acetyl cysteine (NAC) is a supplement that is a precursor to the antioxidant glutathione. Glutathione helps to protect the liver from toxins and damage.

Alpha-lipoic acid is a powerful antioxidant that is found naturally in the body. It is thought to help protect the liver from damage and improve liver function.

Detox Kidneys:

The kidneys are a pair of bean-shaped organs located on either side of the spine, just below the ribcage. They play a crucial role in maintaining overall health by performing several important functions, including filtering the blood to remove waste products and excess fluids, regulating blood pressure, regulating electrolyte balance, and producing hormones. It is important to support kidney health and function to help reduce the risk of kidney-related health problems.

vitamin D and other many nutrients are important for kidney health include potassium, calcium, magnesium and arginine. Potassium helps maintain proper electrolyte balance in the body and Arginine is an amino acid that may help support kidney function and reduce the risk of kidney disease. Bananas are a good source of potassium, with one medium banana providing about 422 milligrams. Nuts and dairy products are good source magnesium and arginine   .Here are several factors that can damage the kidneys and impair their function:

High blood pressure: High blood pressure can damage the blood vessels in the kidneys, leading to kidney damage and reduced function.

Diabetes: High blood sugar levels can damage the blood vessels in the kidneys, leading to kidney damage and reduced function.

Alcohol abuse: Excessive alcohol consumption can impair kidney function and increase the risk of kidney damage.

Infections: Bacterial or viral infections can damage the kidneys and impair their function.

Certain medications: Some medications, such as nonsteroidal anti-inflammatory drugs (NSAIDs) and certain antibiotics, can damage the kidneys and impair their function.

Kidney stones: Kidney stones can block the flow of urine and damage the kidneys.

It is important to manage these risk factors to help reduce the risk of kidney damage and support kidney health. This can include controlling blood pressure and blood sugar levels, avoiding alcohol abuse, getting treatment for infections, drinking paleny of water and using B6 supplements

Supplements that maintain kidneys health and detoxify

Vitamin B6: This vitamin may help support kidney function and reduce the risk of kidney damage.

Chlorella: This type of algae is rich in nutrients and may help support kidney function.

N-acetyl cysteine (NAC): This amino acid may help protect the kidneys from damage and improve kidney function.

Alpha lipoic acid: This antioxidant repair damage and improve kidney function.

6.6 Stress and Aging :

Stress is a normal

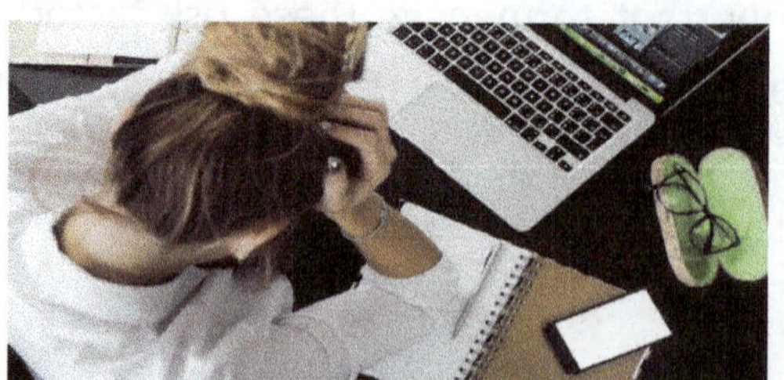

92

response to challenging or demanding situations, but prolonged or chronic stress can have negative effects on overall health. When a person experiences stress, their body releases stress hormones, such as cortisol, which can have physical effects on the body. Stress can affect the immune system, increase the risk of heart disease and other health problems, and cause physical symptoms, such as headaches and difficulty sleeping. Even if a person eats a healthy diet, the negative effects of stress on the body can still contribute to the aging process and overall health problems. It is important to manage stress effectively to support overall health and well-being. This can include practicing relaxation techniques, getting enough sleep, exercising regularly, and seeking support from friends, family, or a healthcare provider.

Here are a few tips that may help you avoid mental stress and be happy in life:

Take care of your physical health: Make sure to get enough sleep, eat a healthy diet, and exercise regularly. These habits can help improve your mood and reduce stress.

Practice mindfulness: This means paying attention to the present moment and being aware of your thoughts and feelings. This can help you gain perspective on your stressors and respond to them more effectively.

Set boundaries: It's important to set limits on your time and energy, and to say no when you need to. This can help prevent you from taking on too much and feeling overwhelmed.

Seek support: Talk to friends and family, or consider finding a therapist or counselor who can help you work through your stressors.

Take breaks: Make time for activities that you enjoy and that help you relax, such as reading, spending time in nature, or practicing a hobby.

Practice gratitude: Taking time to appreciate the good things in your life can help you feel more positive and grateful, which can reduce stress.

Seek out new experiences: Trying new things and stepping out of your comfort zone can help you feel more alive and engaged in life.

There are some supplements that have been shown to have a positive effect on stress and anxiety.

Here are a few examples:

<u>Berries dark chocolates</u>, nuts leafy greens are food that help body reduce stress.

<u>Ashwagandha:</u> Ashwagandha is an herb that has been used for centuries in Ayurvedic medicine to reduce stress and improve overall well-being. Some studies have shown that it may be effective in reducing anxiety and stress.

<u>Magnesium:</u> Magnesium is a mineral that is involved in many bodily processes, including the regulation of stress hormones. Some research suggests that magnesium supplements may be effective in reducing symptoms of anxiety and stress.

<u>B vitamins:</u> B vitamins, particularly B12 and B6, are involved in the production of neurotransmitters that regulate mood. Some research suggests that B vitamin supplements may be helpful in reducing stress and anxiety.

<u>L-theanine:</u> L-theanine is an amino acid that is found in green tea. It has been shown to have a calming effect on the brain and may be effective in reducing stress and anxiety.

How Diabeties and Blood Pressure affects Health

Chapter 7: How Diabetes and Blood Pressure affect Health

Diabetes and high blood pressure are chronic conditions that can have serious effects on the body if not properly managed. These conditions can contribute to the aging process by damaging organs and tissues and increasing the risk of age-related health problems.

A fasting blood sugar level **less than 100 mg/dL (5.6 mmol/L)** is normal. A fasting blood sugar level from 100 to 125 mg/dL (5.6 to 6.9 mmol/L) is considered

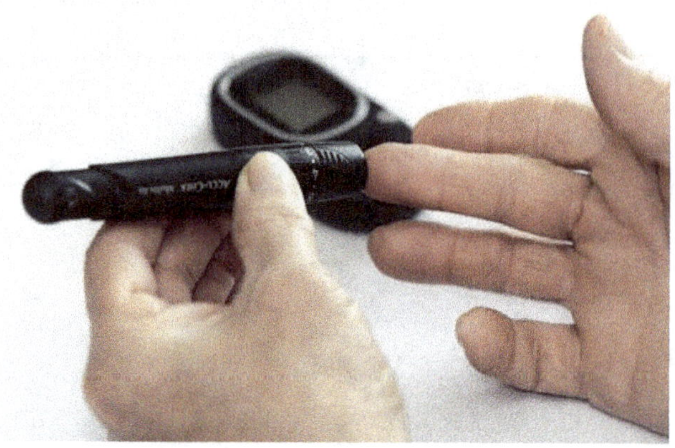

prediabetes. If it's 126 mg/dL (7 mmol/L) or higher on two separate tests, you have diabetes.

If your blood sugar level is too high, you may have:
- Increased thirst
- Frequent urination
- Blurred vision
- Tiredness or weakness
- Headache
- Nausea and vomiting
- Shortness of breath
- Stomach pain
- Fruity breath odor

High blood sugar levels, as seen in diabetes, can damage blood vessels and nerves, leading to a range of complications, including:

Skin problems: High blood sugar levels can affect the skin, leading to dryness, itching, and infections.

Nerve damage: High blood sugar levels can cause nerve damage, leading to numbness, pain, and tingling in the hands, feet, and legs.

Eye problems: High blood sugar levels can cause damage to the blood vessels in the eye, leading to vision loss and blindness.

Kidney damage: High blood sugar levels can damage the blood vessels in the kidneys, leading to kidney damage and reduced function.

Heart disease: People with diabetes have an increased risk of heart disease, including heart attack and stroke.

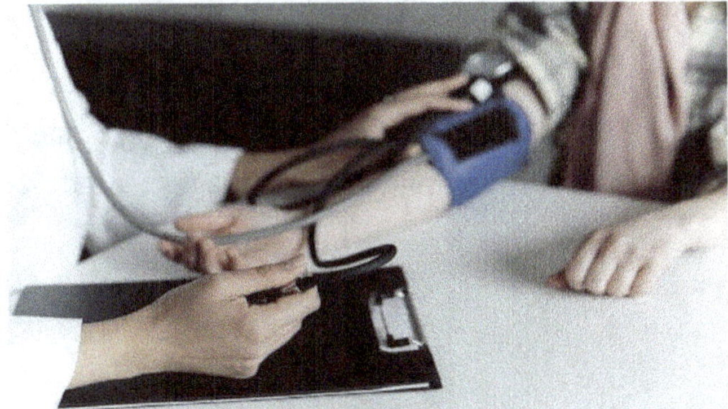

99

High blood pressure can also have serious effects on the body if not properly managed. A normal blood pressure level is **less than 120/80 mmHg**. Some of its symptoms of high blood pressure are:

- Blurred vision.
- Nosebleeds.
- Shortness of breath.
- Chest pain.
- Dizziness.
- Headaches.

High blood pressure can damage blood vessels and increase the risk of a range of complications, including:

Kidney damage: High blood pressure can damage the blood vessels in the kidneys, leading to kidney damage and reduced function.

Heart disease: High blood pressure is a major risk factor for h eart disease. It can damage the blood vessels and increase the risk of plaque build-up, which can lead to heart attack and stroke.

Brain damage: High blood pressure can damage the blood vessels in the brain, leading to a stroke or other brain-related problems.

Overall, both diabetes and high blood pressure can contribute to the aging process by damaging organs and tissues and increasing the risk of age-related health problems. It is important to manage these conditions effectively to help reduce the risk of complications and support overall health. This can include taking medications as prescribed, following a healthy diet and lifestyle, and getting regular medical check-ups.

Chapter 8

Role of Intermittent Fasting in Maintaining Body Health

Chapter 8: Role of Intermittent Fasting in maintaining Body Health

Fasting reduces inflammation in the body by promoting the production of anti-inflammatory substances and decreasing the production of pro-inflammatory substances.

One way that fasting may reduce inflammation is by activating a process called autophagy, which is the body's natural way of cleaning out damaged cells and recycling their components. Autophagy is thought to have a number of important functions in the body, including helping to remove damaged or misfolded proteins, clearing out toxins and waste products, and supporting the immune system.

7.1 Autophagy

Fasting of 16 to 18 hours for a number days is required for triggering autophagy process. Autophagy has been shown to help reduce inflammation and improve the functioning of the

immune system.

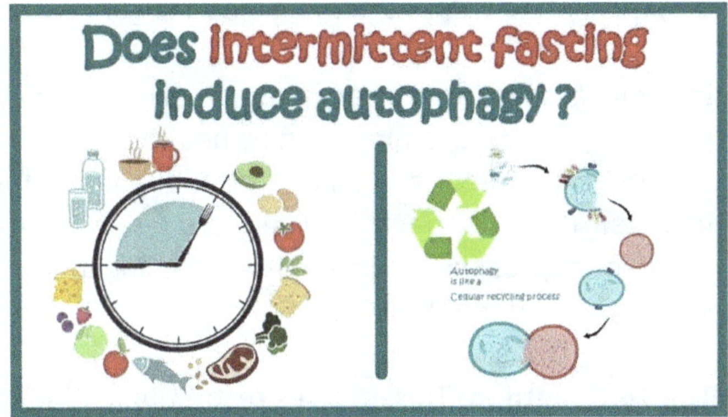

During autophagy, cells identify and target damaged or unnecessary structures, such as proteins, organelles, and other cell components, for degradation.

These materials are then transported to lysosomes, which are organelles that contain enzymes that break down the materials into their component parts. These parts can then be recycled and used to build new, healthy cell components.

8.2 Adiponectin Hormone and Fasting Fasting also has also been shown to increase the production of a hormone called adiponectin, which has anti-inflammatory effects. Adiponectin, an adipokine secreted by adipocytes, is a well-known homeostatic factor for **regulating glucose levels, lipid metabolism, and insulin sensitivity** through its anti-inflammatory, anti-fibrotic, and antioxidant effects. and low levels of adiponectin have been linked to inflammation and a number of chronic diseases.Fating helps regulating blood sugar levels.

Intermittent fasting is a very famous successful way of fasting, being recommended by health experts and researchers of medical sciences round the world for its potential health benefits. There are several different approaches to intermittent fasting, but some common methods include:

The 16/8 method: This involves restricting eating to an 8-hour window each day and fasting for the remaining 16 hours. For example, you might eat all of your meals between noon and 8:00 pm and then fast until noon the next day.

The 5:2 diet: This involves eating normally for 5 days per week and restricting calories to 500-600 per day for the other 2 non-consecutive days.

The alternate-day fasting method: This involves alternating between days of eating normally and days of calorie restriction.

There is some evidence to suggest that intermittent fasting may have a number of potential health benefits, including weight loss, improved insulin sensitivity, and a reduced risk of certain diseases. One can choose the best suitable method.

Chapter 9

Individualized Nutritional Planning

Chapter 9: Individualised Nutritional Planning

9.1 Importance of individualized nutrition planning

Every athlete is unique, with different energy needs, training schedules, and personal preferences. A one-size-fits-all approach to nutrition may not be sufficient for all athletes. Individualized nutrition planning helps athletes meet their specific needs and goals by taking into account factors such as age, gender, body composition, training intensity, and environmental conditions.

Components of Individualized Nutrition Planning

Individualized nutrition planning typically includes the following components:

1: Nutrient needs: Individualized nutrition plans consider an athlete's daily nutrient needs, including macronutrients (carbohydrates, proteins, and fats) and micronutrients (vitamins and minerals). The appropriate balance of these nutrients can help athletes fuel their workouts, support recovery, and optimize performance.

2: Hydration needs: Hydration is an important factor in sports and exercise performance, and individualized nutrition plans take into account an athlete's hydration needs. This may include recommendations for fluid intake before, during, and after exercise, as well as the type of fluid to consume (e.g. water, sports drinks).

3.Meal timing and frequency: Individualized nutrition plans may also consider when and how often an athlete should eat to support their training and recovery. This may include recommendations for pre- and post-exercise meals, as well as strategies for fueling during prolonged exercise.

4. Personal preferences: Individualized nutrition plans take into account an athlete's personal preferences, such as food allergies and intolerances, cultural or dietary restrictions, and taste preferences.

9.2 Benefits of Individualized Nutrition Planning

Individualized nutrition planning offers several benefits for athletes, including:

Improved performance: By meeting an athlete's specific nutrient and hydration needs, individualized nutrition plans can help optimize performance.

Enhanced recovery: Individualized nutrition plans can help athletes refuel and recover effectively after workouts, leading to improved recovery and reduced risk of injury.

Increased energy: Proper nutrition can help athletes feel energized and ready to tackle their workouts.

Improved health: By meeting an athlete's specific nutrient needs, individualized nutrition plans can help support overall health and prevent nutrient deficiencies.

Individualized nutrition planning is an important aspect of sports and exercise performance, providing athletes with a personalized approach to fuel their workouts and support recovery. By taking into account an athlete's unique needs and goals, individualized nutrition plans can help optimize performance and support overall health.

9.3 Three Days customized Plans Examples :

Example 1: Individualized Meal Plan for an Endurance Athlete

Goal: To fuel endurance training and support recovery

Day 1:

Breakfast: Overnight oats with oats, Greek yogurt, berries, and a scoop of protein powder

Snack: Banana and a handful of almonds

Lunch: Grilled chicken salad with mixed greens, cherry tomatoes, and avocado

Snack: Rice cakes with peanut butter and honey

Dinner: Grilled salmon with quinoa and roasted vegetables

Day 2

Breakfast: Scrambled eggs with whole grain toast and spinach

Snack: Apple slices with almond butter

Lunch: Whole grain pasta with tomato sauce, grilled chicken, and roasted vegetables

Snack: Energy bar

Dinner: Grilled tofu with brown rice and steamed broccoli

Day 3:

Breakfast: Oatmeal with sliced bananas, blueberries, and a scoop of protein powder

Snack: Greek yogurt with mixed berries and chia seeds

Lunch: Turkey and avocado wrap with mixed greens and a side of carrot sticks

Snack: Hummus and veggies

Dinner: Grilled steak with sweet potato and roasted asparagus.

Example 2: Individualized Meal Plan for a Weightlifting Athlete

Goal: To build muscle mass and support strength training

Day 1:

Breakfast: Scrambled eggs with whole grain toast and avocado

Snack: Greek yogurt with mixed berries and a scoop of protein powder

Lunch: Grilled chicken with quinoa and roasted vegetables

Snack: Hard boiled egg and a handful of almonds

Dinner: Grilled steak with sweet potato and broccoli

Day 2:

Breakfast: Overnight oats with oats, Greek yogurt, berries, and a scoop of protein powder

Snack: Banana and peanut butter.

Lunch: Turkey and avocado wrap with mixed greens and a side of carrot sticks

Snack: Rice cakes with hummus and sliced veggies

Dinner: Grilled tofu with brown rice and steamed broccoli

Day 3

Breakfast: Scrambled eggs with whole grain toast and spinach

Snack: Apple slices with almond butter

Lunch: Whole grain pasta with tomato sauce, grilled chicken, and roasted vegetables

Snack: Energy bar

Dinner: Grilled salmon with quinoa and roasted vegetables

This meal plan includes a balance of protein and carbohydrates to support muscle growth and recovery. It also includes a variety of whole, unprocessed foods to provide the necessary nutrients for strength training.

Individualized meal plan for weight loss and muscle gain

Example: Individualized Meal Plan for Weight Loss and Muscle Gain

Goal: To lose weight and build muscle mass

Day 1:

Breakfast: Scrambled eggs with whole grain toast and avocado

Snack: Greek yogurt with mixed berries and a scoop of protein powder

Lunch: Grilled chicken with quinoa and roasted vegetables

Snack: Hard boiled egg and a handful of almonds

Dinner: Grilled steak with sweet potato and broccoli

Day 2:

Breakfast: Overnight oats with oats, Greek yogurt, berries, and a scoop of protein powder

Snack: Banana and peanut butter

Lunch: Turkey and avocado wrap with mixed greens and a side of carrot sticks

Snack: Rice cakes with hummus and sliced veggies

Dinner: Grilled tofu with brown rice and steamed broccoli

Day 3:

Breakfast: Scrambled eggs with whole grain toast and spinach

Snack: Apple slices with almond butter

Lunch: Whole grain pasta with tomato sauce, grilled chicken, and roasted vegetables

Snack: Energy bar

Dinner: Grilled salmon with quinoa and roasted vegetables

This meal plans include a balance of protein and carbohydrates to support muscle growth and recovery, while also limiting calories to support weight loss. It also includes a variety of whole, unprocessed foods to provide the necessary nutrients for muscle gain and weight loss. It is important to note that this meal plan is just an example and that individualized nutrition planning is important to ensure that an athlete's specific needs and goals are met.

9.3 Recipes of Healthy Snacking and Meals

Here are five healthy snack recipes that are rich in protein:

Peanut Butter Energy Bites: In a medium bowl, mix together the oats, peanut butter, flaxseed, and chocolate chips.
Add the honey and vanilla extract and mix until well combined. 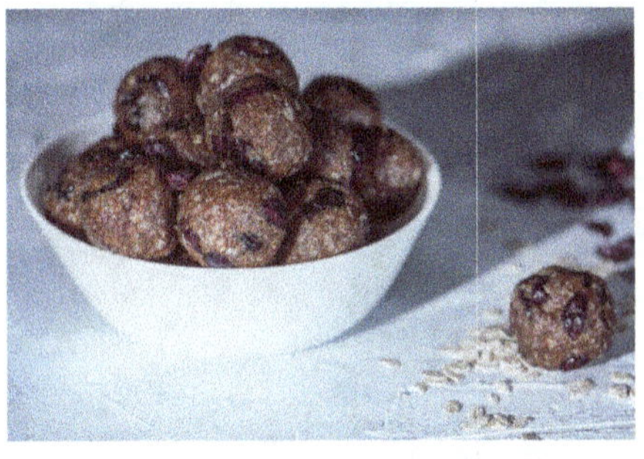
Roll the mixture into balls, about 1 inch in diameter. Place the balls on a plate or baking sheet and refrigerate until firm, about 1 hour.

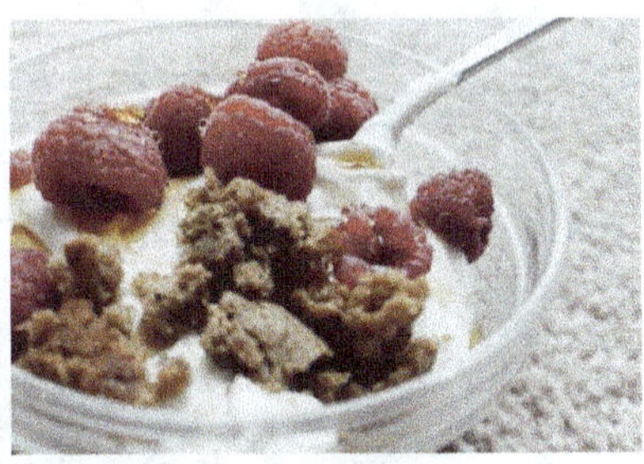

Greek Yogurt Parfait: Combine 1 cup Greek yogurt with 1/2 cup mixed berries and 1/4 cup granola. Layer the ingredients in a jar or glass and enjoy as a delicious and protein-rich snack.

Hummus and Veggie Sticks: Dip carrot, celery, or bell pepper sticks into a small bowl of hummus for a protein-rich snack.

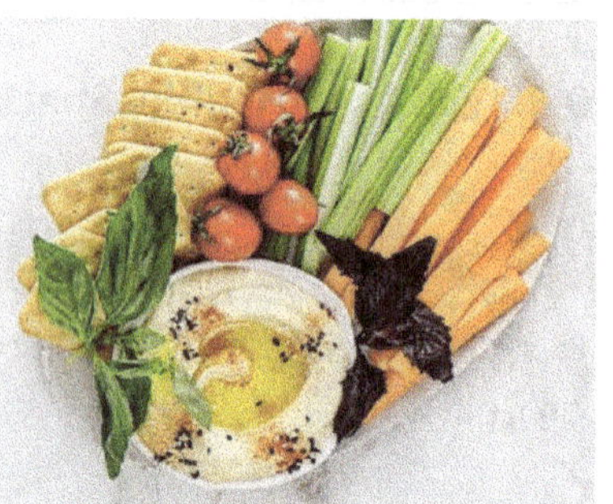

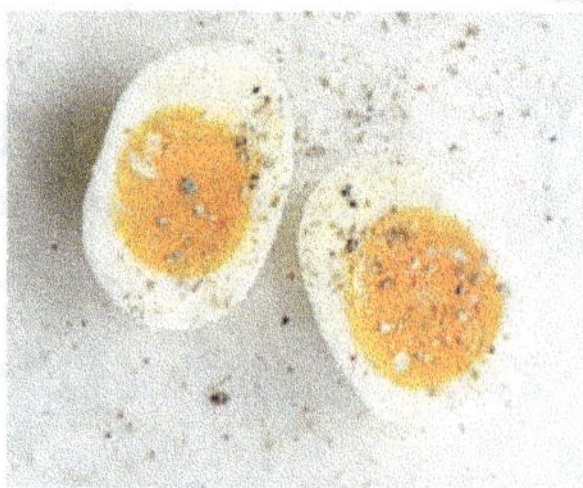

Hard-Boiled Eggs: Hard-boiled eggs are a convenient and protein-rich snack that can be easily packed and taken on the go.

Healthy meals Examples

Baked Salmon with Roasted Vegetables:

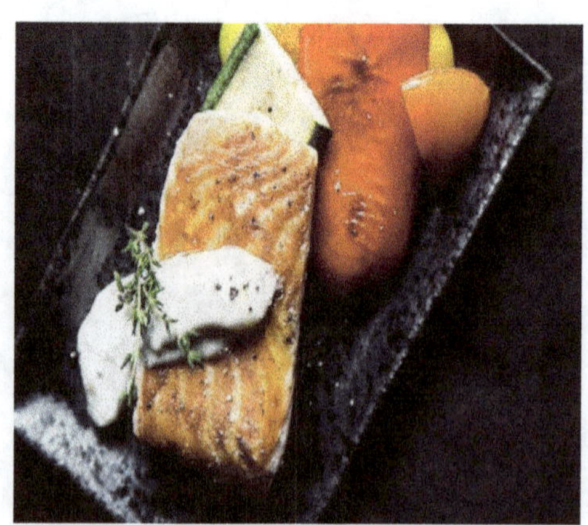

Ingredients: 4 salmon fillets, 1 cup mixed vegetables (such as broccoli, bell peppers, and carrots), 2 tbsp olive oil, Salt and pepper, to taste, 2 tbsp cheese

Instructions:

Preheat the oven to 400°F (200°C).

Place the salmon fillets in a baking dish.

In a separate bowl, toss the vegetables with the olive oil, salt, and pepper. Arrange the vegetables around the salmon in the baking dish.Bake for 15-20 minutes, or until the salmon is cooked through and the vegetables are tender.

Sprinkle the cheese over the top of the salmon and vegetables and bake for an additional 5 minutes, or until the cheese is melted.

Grilled Chicken with Caesar Salad:

Ingredients: 4 chicken breasts, 2 tbsp olive oil, Salt and pepper, to

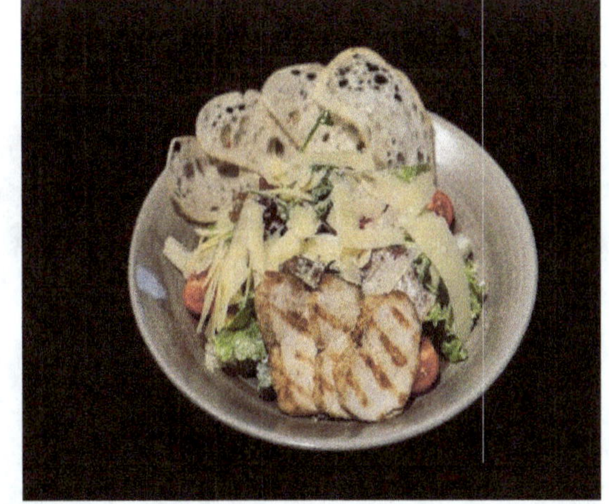

taste, 4 cups mixed greens, 1/2 cup Caesar dressing, 1/4 cup grated Parmesan cheese

Instructions:

1. Preheat the grill to medium-high heat.
2. Brush the chicken breasts with olive oil and season with salt and pepper.
3. Grill the chicken for 6-8 minutes on each side, or until cooked through.
4. In a large bowl, toss the mixed greens with the Caesar dressing.
5. Divide the salad among four plates and top with the grilled chicken.
6. Sprinkle the Parmesan cheese over the top and serve.

Quinoa and Black Bean Salad with Nuts and Seeds

Ingredients:

- 1 cup quinoa
- 2 cups water
- 1 can black beans, drained and rinsed
- 1 bell pepper, diced
- 1 cup cherry tomatoes, halved
- 1/2 cup diced red onion

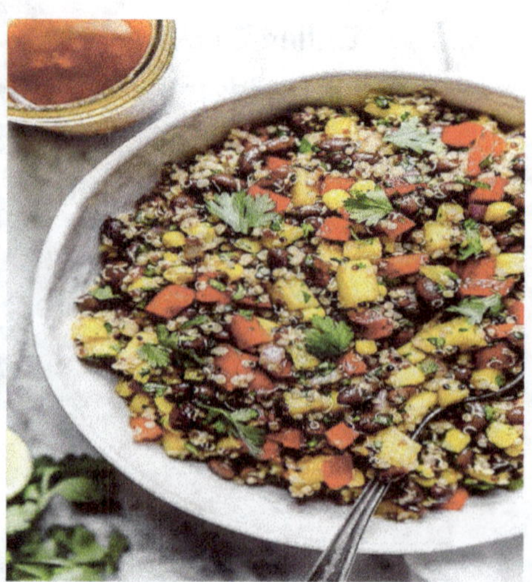

- 1/2 cup chopped fresh cilantro
- 2 tablespoons olive oil
- 2 tablespoons lemon juice
- 1 clove garlic, minced
- Salt and pepper, to taste
- 1/2 cup mixed nuts and seeds (such as almonds, sunflower seeds, and pumpkin seeds)

Instructions:

1. Rinse the quinoa in a fine mesh strainer. In a medium saucepan, bring the quinoa and water to a boil. Reduce the heat to low, cover, and simmer for 15-20 minutes, or until the quinoa is cooked and the water has been absorbed.
2. In a large bowl, combine the cooked quinoa, black beans, bell pepper, cherry tomatoes, red onion, and cilantro.
3. In a small bowl, whisk together the olive oil, lemon juice, and garlic. Season with salt and pepper to taste. Pour the dressing over the quinoa mixture and toss to coat.
4. Toast the nuts and seeds in a dry pan over medium heat until fragrant and lightly browned.
5. Serve the quinoa and black bean salad topped with the toasted nuts and seeds. Enjoy!